Keto Diet Cookbook for Women After 50

An Effective Guide to Uncovering Boundless Energy and Your Happy Weight. Mouthwatering Low-Carb Recipes to Face Menopause Without Stress, Reset Metabolism and Stay Healthy

Written By

Claire Goldenpond

Table of Contents

INTRODUCTION

Thank you for purchasing this book!

Compounding these issues is that as we age, our bodies require less fuel, and we need to decrease the number of calories we eat in a day. This makes it challenging to make sure we get the nutrients needed while eating fewer calories. It's a bit of a nutritional dilemma.

Lucky for us, there are several steps you can do to prevent deficiencies and other age-related changes. As an example, consuming food that is rich in nutrients and ingesting the right supplements can aid in keeping you healthy as you age. Following a Keto-diet is one great way of staying healthy as you continue to age.

Enjoy your reading!

BREAKFAST

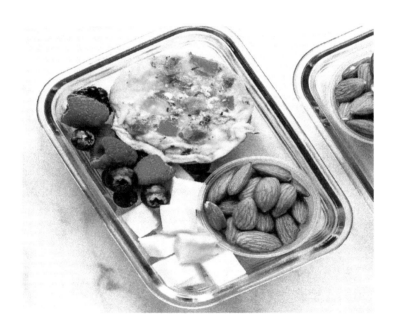

Coconut Keto Porridge

Preparation Time: 15 minutes

Cooking Time: 10 minutes

Servings: 2

Ingredients:

- 4 tbsp. coconut cream
- 1 pinch ground psyllium husk powder
- 1 tbsp. coconut flour
- 1 flaxseed egg
- 1oz. coconut butter

Directions:

1. Toss all of the mixtures in a small pan, cook on low heat. Serve.

Nutrition:

- Net Carbohydrates: 5.4 g
- Protein: 10.1 g
- Fat: 22.8 g
- Calories: 401

Mexican Scrambled Eggs

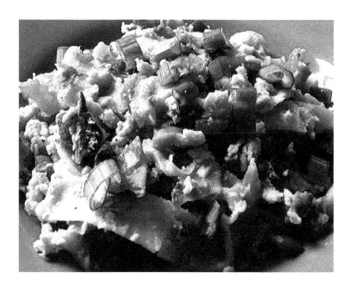

Preparation Time: 5 minutes

Cooking Time: 5 minutes

Servings: 2

Ingredients:

- 1/2 tsp salt
- 3 eggs
- 1/2 scallion, chopped
- 1/2 medium tomato, chopped
- 1 pickled jalapeño, chopped
- 1 ½ oz. shredded cheddar cheese
- 1 tbsp butter
- 1/2 tsp salt
- ½ tsp ground black pepper

Directions:

1. Place a large skillet pan over medium-high heat, add butter and when it melts, add scallion, tomato, and jalapeno and cook for 3 minutes or until beginning to soften.
2. Meanwhile, crack eggs in a bowl and whisk until beaten.
3. Pour the egg mixture into the pan, scramble eggs for 2 minutes, then sprinkle cheese on top and season with salt and black pepper.
4. Serve straight away.

Nutrition:

- Net Carbohydrates: 2g
- Protein: 14g
- Fat: 12g
- Calories: 229

Coconut Porridge

Preparation Time: 5 minutes

Cooking Time: 10 minutes

Servings: 2

Ingredients

- 2 eggs, beaten
- 2 tbsp coconut flour
- 1/8 tsp. salt
- 1/8 tsp. psyllium husk powder grounded
- 2 oz. butter
- 8 tbsp coconut cream

Directions:

1. Crack eggs in a bowl, add flour, salt, and Psyllium husk, and whisk until combined.
2. Place a saucepan over low heat, add butter and when it melts, whisk in coconut cream.
3. Then slowly whisk in egg mixture until a smooth and creamy mixture comes together.
4. Divide porridge evenly between two bowls and serve with berries.

Nutrition:

- Net Carbohydrates: 4g
- Protein: 9g
- Fat: 49g
- Calories: 486

Cauliflower Hash Browns

Preparation Time: 10 minutes

Cooking Time: 30 minutes

Servings: 2

Ingredients:

- ½ lb. cauliflower, grated
- 2 eggs
- ¼ white onion, grated
- ½ tsp salt
- ¼ tsp ground black pepper
- 2 oz. butter, for frying

Directions:

1. Place grated cauliflower in a bowl, add remaining ingredients and stir until mixed, let the mixture rest for 10 minutes.
2. Then place a skillet pan over medium heat, add butter and when it melts, lower the heat and place scoops of the cauliflower mixture.
3. Flatten each mixture into 3 to 4-inch patties and fry for 4 to 5 minutes per side or until nicely golden brown and cooked.
4. Serve straight away.

Nutrition:

- Net Carbohydrates: 5g
- Protein: 7g
- Fat: 26g
- Calories: 282

Cream Cheese Eggs

Preparation Time: 5 minutes

Cooking Time: 5 minutes

Servings: 2

Ingredients:

- 1 tbsp. Butter
- 2 Eggs
- 2 tbsp. Soft cream cheese with chives

Directions:

1. Warm-up a skillet and melt the butter. Whisk the eggs with the cream cheese.
2. Cook until done. Serve.

Nutrition:

- Net Carbohydrates: 3 g
- Protein: 15 g
- Fat: 31 g
- Calories: 341

SOUPS & FIRST COURSES

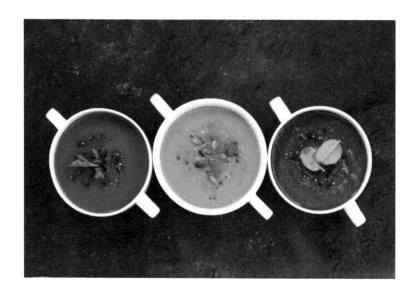

Quinoa Salad with Fresh Mint and Parsley

Preparation Time: 10 minutes

Cooking Time: 15 minutes

Servings: 2

Ingredients:

- 2 cups of quinoa
- 1/2 cup of almond nut
- 3 tbsp. of fresh parsley (chopped)
- 1/2 cup of chopped green onions
- 3 tbsp. of chopped fresh mint
- 3 tbsp. of olive oil
- 2 tbsp. of lemon juice
- 1 tsp. of garlic salt
- 1/2 tsp. of salt and pepper

Directions:

1. Place a saucepan on high heat.
2. Add the quinoa and water and just let it boil for around 15 minutes, then reduce the heat and drain.
3. Pour the drained quinoa into a large bowl, add the parsley, almond nuts, and mint.
4. In a bowl or container, add the olive oil, garlic salt, and lemon juice together.
5. Whisk the mixture well until it's well combined and pour over the quinoa.

6. Combine the mixture well until everything is well dispersed.
7. Add the salt and black pepper to taste.
8. Place the quinoa mixture bowl in the refrigerator.

Nutrition:

- Net Carbohydrates: 2.1 g
- Protein: 9.3g
- Fat: 8.4g
- Calories: 241

Coconut Soup

Preparation Time: 15 minutes

Cooking Time: 35 minutes

Servings: 2

Ingredients:

- 1½ cups of coconut milk
- 4 cups chicken stock
- 1 tsp fried lemongrass
- 3 lime leaves
- 4 Thai chilies, dried and chopped
- 1-inch fresh ginger, peeled and grated
- 1 cup fresh cilantro, chopped
- Salt and ground black pepper to taste
- 1 tbsp fish sauce
- 1 tbsp coconut oil
- 2 tbsp mushrooms, chopped
- 4 oz shrimp, peeled and deveined
- 2 tbsp onion, chopped
- 1 tbsp fresh cilantro, chopped
- Juice from 1 lime

Directions:

1. In a medium pot, combine coconut milk, chicken stock, lemongrass, and lime leaves.
2. Preheat the pot on medium heat.

3. Add Thai chilies, ginger, cilantro, salt, and pepper, stir and bring to simmer—Cook for 20 minutes.
4. Strain the soup and return liquid to the pot.
5. Heat the soup over medium heat.
6. Add fish sauce, coconut oil, mushrooms, shrimp, and onion. Stir well—Cook for 10 minutes.
7. Add cilantro and lime juice, stir. Set aside for 10 minutes.
8. Serve.

Nutrition:

- Net Carbohydrates: 7.9g
- Protein: 11.8g
- Fat: 33.8g
- Calories: 448

Broccoli Soup

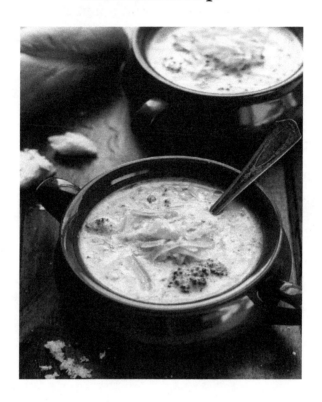

Preparation Time: 12 minutes

Cooking Time: 35 minutes

Servings: 2

Ingredients:

- 2 cloves garlic
- 1 medium white onion
- 1 tbsp butter
- 2 cups of water
- 2 cups vegetable stock

- 1 cup heavy cream
- Salt and ground black pepper to taste
- ½ tsp paprika
- 1½ cups broccoli, divided into florets
- 1 cup cheddar cheese

Directions:

1. Peel and mince garlic. Peel and chop the onion.
2. Preheat the pot on medium heat, add butter and melt it.
3. Add garlic and onion and sauté for 5 minutes, stirring occasionally.
4. Pour in water, vegetable stock, heavy cream, and add pepper, salt, and paprika.
5. Stir and bring to a boil.
6. Add broccoli and simmer for 25 minutes.
7. After that, transfer the soup mixture to a food processor and blend well.
8. Grate cheddar cheese and add to a food processor, blend again.
9. Serve soup hot.

Nutrition:

- Net Carbohydrates: 6.8g
- Protein: 10.9g
- Fat: 33.8g
- Calories: 348

Simple Tomato Soup

Preparation Time: 15 minutes

Cooking Time: 10 minutes

Servings: 2

Ingredients:

- 4 cups canned tomato soup
- 2 tbsp apple cider vinegar
- 1 tsp dried oregano
- 4 tbsp butter
- 2 tsp turmeric
- 2 oz red hot sauce
- Salt and ground black pepper to taste
- 4 tbsp olive oil
- 8 bacon strips, cooked and crumbled
- 4 oz fresh basil leaves, chopped
- 4 oz green onions, chopped

Directions:

1. Pour tomato soup into the pot and preheat on medium heat. Bring to a boil.
2. Add vinegar, oregano, butter, turmeric, hot sauce, salt, black pepper, and olive oil. Stir well.
3. Simmer the soup for 5 minutes.
4. Serve soup topped with crumbled bacon, green onion, and basil.

Nutrition:

- Net Carbohydrates: 9g
- Protein: 11.7g
- Fat: 33.8
- Calories: 397

<u>Green Soup</u>

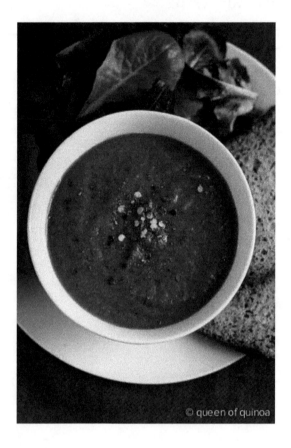

Preparation Time: 12 minutes

Cooking Time: 15 minutes

Servings: 2

Ingredients:

- 2 cloves garlic
- 1 white onion
- 1 cauliflower head

- 2 oz butter
- 1 bay leaf, crushed
- 1 cup spinach leaves
- ½ cup watercress
- 4 cups vegetable stock
- Salt and ground black pepper to taste
- 1 cup of coconut milk
- ½ cup parsley for serving

Directions:

1. Peel and mince garlic. Peel and dice onion.
2. Divide cauliflower into florets.
3. Preheat the pot on medium-high heat, add butter and melt it.
4. Add onion and garlic, stir, and sauté for 4 minutes.
5. Add cauliflower and bay leaf, stir and cook for 5 minutes.
6. Add spinach and watercress, stir and cook for another 3 minutes.
7. Pour in vegetable stock—season with salt and black pepper. Stir and bring to a boil.
8. Pour in coconut milk and stir well. Take off heat.
9. Use an immersion blender to blend well.
10. Top with parsley and serve hot.

Nutrition:

- Net Carbohydrates: 4.89g
- Protein: 6.97g
- Fat: 35.1
- Calories: 227

Sausage and Peppers Soup

Preparation Time: 15 minutes

Cooking Time: 1 hour 15 minutes

Servings: 2

Ingredients:

- 1 tbsp avocado oil
- 2 lbs. pork sausage meat
- Salt and ground black pepper to taste
- 1 green bell pepper, seeded and chopped
- 5 oz canned jalapeños, chopped
- 5 oz canned tomatoes, chopped
- 1¼ cup spinach
- 4 cups beef stock
- 1 tsp Italian seasoning
- 1 tbsp cumin
- 1 tsp onion powder
- 1 tsp garlic powder
- 1 tbsp chili powder

Directions:

1. Preheat pot with avocado oil on medium heat.
2. Put sausage meat in pot and brown for 3 minutes on all sides.
3. Add salt, black pepper, and green bell pepper and continue to cook for 3 minutes.

4. Add jalapeños and tomatoes, stir well, and cook for 2 minutes more.

5. Toss spinach and stir again, close the lid and cook for 7 minutes.

6. Pour in beef stock, Italian seasoning, cumin, onion powder, chili powder, garlic powder, salt, and black pepper, stir well. Close lid again. Cook for 30 minutes.

7. When time is up, uncover the pot and simmer for 15 minutes more.

8. Serve hot.

Nutrition:

- Net Carbohydrates: 3.99g
- Protein: 25.8g
- Fat: 44.5g
- Calories: 531

FISH & SEAFOOD

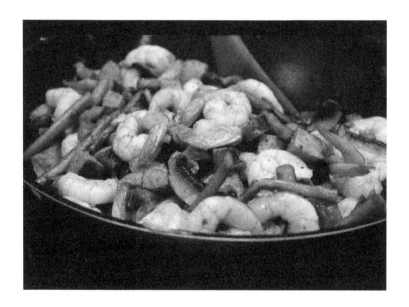

Turmeric Tilapia

Preparation Time: 10 minutes

Cooking Time: 12 minutes

Servings: 2

Ingredients:

- 4 tilapia fillets, boneless
- 2 tbsp. olive oil
- 1 tsp. turmeric powder
- A pinch of salt and black pepper
- 2 spring onions, chopped
- ¼ tsp. basil, dried
- ¼ tsp. garlic powder
- 1 tbsp. parsley, chopped

Directions:

1. Heat a pan with the oil over medium heat, add the spring onions and cook them for 2 minutes.
2. Add the fish, turmeric, and the other ingredients, cook for 5 minutes on each side, divide between plates and serve.

Nutrition:

- Net Carbohydrates: 1.1g
- Protein: 31.8 g
- Fat: 8.6g
- Calories: 205

Walnut Salmon Mix

Preparation Time: 10 minutes

Cooking Time: 14 minutes

Servings: 2

Ingredients:

- 2 salmon fillets, boneless
- 2 tbsp. avocado oil
- A pinch of salt and black pepper
- 1 tbsp. lime juice
- 2 shallots, chopped
- 2 tbsp. walnuts, chopped
- 2 tbsp. parsley, chopped

Directions:

1. Heat a pan with the oil over medium-high heat, add the shallots, stir and sauté for 2 minutes.
2. Add the fish and the other ingredients, cook for 6 minutes on each side, divide between plates and serve.

Nutrition:

- Net Carbohydrates: 2.7g
- Protein: 35.8 g
- Fat: 14.2g
- Calories: 276

Cioppino

Preparation Time: 15 minutes

Cooking Time: 30 minutes

Servings: 2

Ingredients:

- 2 tbsp. olive oil
- 1/2 onion, chopped
- 2 celery stalks, sliced
- 1 red bell pepper, chopped
- 1 tbsp. minced garlic
- 2 cups fish stock
- 1 (15-oz.) can coconut milk
- 1 cup crushed tomatoes
- 2 tbsp. tomato paste
- 1 tbsp. chopped fresh basil
- 2 tsp. chopped fresh oregano
- 1/2 tsp. of sea salt
- 1/2 tsp. freshly ground black pepper
- 1/4 tsp. red pepper flakes
- 10 oz. salmon, cut into 1-inch pieces
- 1/2 lb. shrimp, peeled and deveined
- 12 clams or mussels, cleaned and debearded but in the shell

Directions:

1. Sauté the vegetables.
2. In a pot, warm the olive oil. Add the onion, celery, red bell pepper, and garlic and sauté until they've softened about 4 minutes.
3. Make the soup base. Stir in the fish stock, coconut milk, crushed tomatoes, tomato paste, basil, oregano, salt, pepper, and red pepper flakes.
4. Boil and then simmer the soup for 10 minutes.
5. Add the seafood. Stir in the salmon and simmer until it goes opaque, about 5 minutes.
6. Add the shrimp and simmer until they're almost cooked through about 3 minutes. Add the mussels.
7. Serve.

Nutrition:

- Net Carbohydrates: 4.2 g
- Protein: 16.4g
- Fat: 11.1g
- Calories: 321

Coconut Mussels

Preparation Time: 10 minutes

Cooking Time: 10-15 minutes

Servings: 2

Ingredients:

- 2 tbsp. coconut oil
- 1/2 sweet onion, chopped
- 2 tsp. minced garlic
- 1 tsp. grated fresh ginger
- 1/2 tsp. turmeric
- 1 cup of coconut milk
- Juice of 1 lime
- 1 1/2 lb. fresh mussels, scrubbed and debearded
- 1 scallion, finely chopped
- 2 tbsp. chopped fresh cilantro
- 1 tbsp. chopped fresh thyme

Directions:

1. Sauté the aromatics.
2. In a pot, warm the coconut oil. Add the onion, garlic, ginger, and turmeric and sauté until they've softened about 3 minutes.
3. Add the liquid. Stir in the coconut milk and lime juice and bring the mixture to a boil.
4. Steam the mussels.

5. Add the mussels to the skillet, cover, and steam until the shells are open, about 10 minutes.
6. Take the skillet off the heat and throw out any unopened mussels.
7. Add the herbs. Stir in the scallion, cilantro, and thyme.
8. Divide the mussels and the sauce between four bowls and serve them immediately.

Nutrition:

- Net Carbohydrates: 1.2 g
- Protein: 1.4g
- Fat: 11.1g
- Calories: 321

Italian Style Halibut Packets

Preparation Time: 10 minutes

Cooking Time: 20 minutes

Servings: 2

Ingredients:

- 2 cups cauliflower florets
- 1 cup roasted red pepper strips
- 1/2 cup sliced sun-dried tomatoes
- 4 (4-oz.) halibut fillets
- 1/4 cup chopped fresh basil
- Juice of 1 lemon
- 1/4 cup good-quality olive oil
- Sea salt for seasoning
- Freshly ground black pepper for seasoning

Directions:

1. Preheat the oven. Set the oven temperature to 400°F.
2. Make the packets.
3. Divide the cauliflower, red pepper strips, and sun-dried tomato between the four pieces of foil, placing the vegetables in the middle of each piece.
4. Top each pile with one halibut fillet, and top each fillet with equal amounts of basil, lemon juice, and olive oil.
5. Fold and crimp the foil to form sealed packets of fish and vegetables and place them on the baking sheet.

6. Bake the packets for about 20 minutes, until the fish flakes with a fork.
7. Be careful of the steam when you open the packet!
8. Transfer the vegetables and halibut to four plates, season with salt and pepper, and serve immediately.

Nutrition:

- Net Carbohydrates: 3.2 g
- Protein: 15.4g
- Fat: 14.1g
- Calories: 313

Greek Tuna Salad

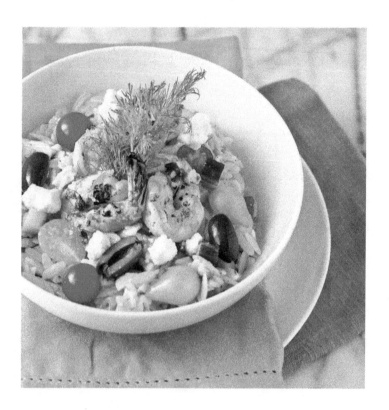

Preparation Time: 10 minutes

Cooking Time: 0 minutes

Servings: 2

Ingredients:

- 3 cans of tuna
- 1/4 small red onion, finely chopped
- 1 celery stalks, finely chopped
- 1/2 avocado, chopped
- 1 tbsp. chopped fresh parsley

- 1 cup Greek yogurt
- 2 tbsp. butter
- 2 tsp. Dijon Mustard
- 1/2 tbsp. vinegar
- Salt and black pepper to taste

Directions:

1. The ingredients listed must be added to a salad bowl and mix until well combined.
2. Serve afterward.

Nutrition:

- Net Carbohydrates: 3.9 g
- Protein: 18.4g
- Fat: 10.4g
- Calories: 376

Blackened Salmon with Avocado Salsa

Preparation Time: 15 minutes

Cooking Time: 10 minutes

Servings: 2

Ingredients:

- 1 tbsp. extra virgin olive oil
- 2 filets of salmon (about 6 oz. each)
- 2 tsp. Cajun seasoning
- 1 med. avocados, diced
- 1 c. cucumber, diced
- 1/4 c. red onion, diced
- 1 tbsp. parsley, chopped
- 1 tbsp. lime juice
- Sea salt & pepper to taste

Directions:

1. The oil must be heated in a skillet.
2. Rub the Cajun seasoning into the fillets, then lay them into the bottom of the skillet once it's hot enough.
3. Cook until a dark crust forms, then flip and repeat.
4. In a medium mixing bowl, combine all the ingredients for the salsa and set aside.
5. Plate the fillets and top with 1/4 of the salsa yielded.
6. Enjoy!

Nutrition:

- Net Carbohydrates: 4.1 g
- Protein: 11.8g
- Fat: 15.8g
- Calories: 425

Tangy Coconut Cod

Preparation Time: 10 minutes

Cooking Time: 10 minutes

Servings: 2

Ingredients:

- 1/3 c. coconut flour
- 1/2 tsp. cayenne pepper
- 1 egg, beaten
- 1 lime
- 1 tsp. crushed red pepper flakes
- 1 tsp. garlic powder
- 12 oz. cod fillets
- Sea salt & pepper to taste

Directions:

1. Let the oven preheat to 400°F/175°C. Then line a baking sheet with non-stick foil.
2. Place the flour in a shallow dish (a plate works fine) and drag the fillets of cod through the beaten egg. Dredge the cod in the coconut flour, then lay it on the baking sheet.
3. Sprinkle top of steak with seasoning and lemon juice.
4. Bake the cod for about 10 to 12 minutes until the fillets are flaky.
5. Serve immediately!

Nutrition:

- Net Carbohydrates: 4.1 g
- Protein: 19.5g
- Fat: 12.1g
- Calories: 318

BEEF, PORK & LAMB

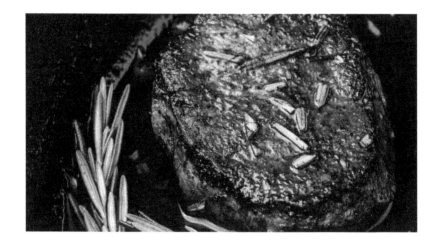

Lamb Chops with Tapenade

Preparation Time: 15 minutes

Cooking Time: 25 minutes

Servings: 2

Ingredients:

For the Tapenade:

- 1 cup pitted Kalamata olive
- 2 tbsp. chopped fresh parsley
- 2 tbsp. extra-virgin olive oil
- 2 tsp. minced garlic
- 2 tsp. freshly squeezed lemon juice

For the Lamb Chops:

- 2 (1-lb.) racks French-cut lamb chops (8 bones each)
- Sea salt
- Freshly ground black pepper
- 1 tbsp. olive oil

Directions:

To Make The Tapenade:

1. Place the olives, parsley, olive oil, garlic, and lemon juice in a food processor and process until the mixture is puréed but still slightly chunky.
2. Transfer the tapenade to a container and store it sealed in the refrigerator until needed.

To Make The Lamb Chops:

1. Preheat the oven to 450°F.

2. Season the lamb racks with pepper and salt

3. Heat oil.

4. Pan sear the lamb racks on all sides until browned, about 5 minutes in total.

5. Arrange the racks upright in the skillet, with the bones interlaced, and roast them for about 20 minutes for medium-rare or until the internal temperature reaches 125°F.

Nutrition:

- Net Carbohydrates: 5.4 g
- Protein: 18.9g
- Fat: 17.4g
- Calories: 387

Sesame Pork with Green Beans

Preparation Time: 5 minutes

Cooking Time: 10 minutes

Servings: 2

Ingredients:

- 2 boneless pork chops
- Pink Himalayan salt
- Freshly ground black pepper
- 2 tbsp. toasted sesame oil, divided
- 2 tbsp. soy sauce
- 1 tsp. Sriracha sauce
- 1 cup fresh green beans

Directions:

1. On a cutting board, pat the pork chops dry with a paper towel. Slice the chops into strips and season with pink Himalayan salt and pepper.
2. In a large skillet over medium heat, heat one tbsp. of sesame oil.
3. Add the pork strips and cook them for 7 minutes, stirring occasionally.
4. In a small bowl, mix the remaining one tbsp. of sesame oil, soy sauce, and Sriracha sauce. Pour into the skillet with the pork.
5. Add the green beans to the skillet, reduce the heat to medium-low, and simmer for 3 to 5 minutes.

6. Divide the pork, green beans, and sauce between two wide, shallow bowls and serve.

Nutrition:

- Net Carbohydrates: 4.1 g
- Protein:18.1 g
- Fat: 15.1g
- Calories: 387

Garlicky Prime Rib Roast

Preparation Time: 15 minutes

Cooking Time: 1 hour 35 minutes

Servings: 2

Ingredients:

- 5 garlic cloves
- 2 tsp. dried thyme
- 2 tbsp. olive oil
- Salt
- ground black pepper
- 1 grass-fed prime rib roast

Directions:

1. Mix the garlic, thyme, oil, salt, and black pepper. Marinate the rib roast with garlic mixture for 1 hour.
2. Warm-up oven to 500 degrees F.
3. Roast for 20 minutes. Lower to 325 degrees F and roast for 65-75 minutes.
4. Remove then chill in 10-15 minutes, slice, and serve.

Nutrition:

- Protein: 61.5g
- Fat: 25.9g
- Calories: 499

Beef Taco Bake

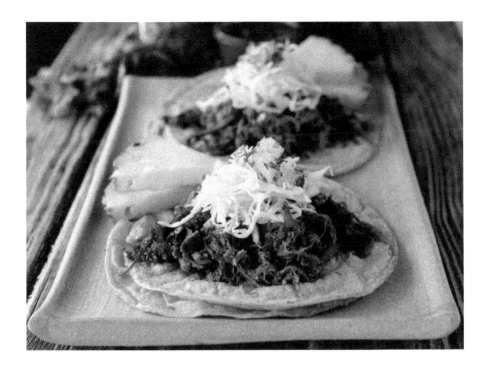

Preparation Time: 15 minutes

Cooking Time: 1 hour

Servings: 2

Ingredients:

For Crust:

- 3 organic eggs
- 4 oz. cream cheese
- ½ tsp. taco seasoning
- 1/3 cup heavy cream
- 8 oz. cheddar cheese

For Topping:

- 1-lb. grass-fed ground beef
- 4 oz. green chilies
- ¼ cup sugar-free tomato sauce
- 3 tsp. taco seasoning
- 8 oz. cheddar cheese

Directions:

1. Warm-up oven to 375 degrees F.
2. For the crust: beat the eggs, and cream cheese, taco seasoning, and heavy cream.
3. Place cheddar cheese in the baking dish. Spread cream cheese mixture over cheese.
4. Bake for 25-30 minutes. Remove and then set aside for 5 minutes.

For topping:

1. Cook the beef for 8-10 minutes.
2. Stir in the green chilies, tomato sauce, and taco seasoning and transfer.
3. Place the beef mixture over the crust and sprinkle with cheese. Bake for 18-20 minutes.
4. Remove and then slice and serve.

Nutrition:

- Net Carbohydrates: 4g
- Protein: 38.7g
- Fat: 23g
- Calories: 569

Meatballs Curry

Preparation Time: 15 minutes

Cooking Time: 25 minutes

Servings: 2

Ingredients

For Meatballs:

- 1-lb. lean ground pork
- 2 organic eggs
- 3 tbsp. yellow onion
- ¼ cup fresh parsley leaves
- ¼ tsp. fresh ginger
- 2 garlic cloves
- 1 jalapeño pepper
- 1 tsp. Erythritol
- 1 tbsp. red curry paste
- 3 tbsp. olive oil

For Curry:

- 1 yellow onion
- Salt
- 2 garlic cloves
- ¼ tsp. ginger
- 2 tbsp. red curry paste
- 1 can unsweetened coconut milk
- Ground black pepper

- ¼ cup fresh parsley

Directions:

For meatballs:

1. Mix all the ingredients except oil. Make small-sized balls from the mixture.
2. Cook meatballs for 3-5 minutes. Transfer and put aside.

For curry:

1. Sauté onion and salt for 4-5 minutes. Add the garlic and ginger. Add the curry paste, and sauté for 1-2 minutes. Add coconut milk and meatballs then simmer.
2. Simmer again for 10-12 minutes. Put salt and black pepper. Remove then serve with fresh parsley.

Nutrition:

- Net Carbohydrates: 6.4g
- Protein: 17g
- Fat: 31g
- Calories: 444

POULTRY & EGGS

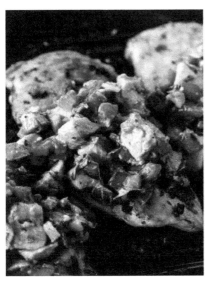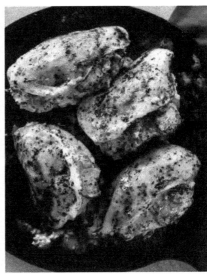

Chili Lime Chicken with Coleslaw

Preparation Time: 35 minutes

Cooking Time: 8 minutes

Servings: 2

Ingredients:

- 1 chicken thigh, boneless
- 2 oz. coleslaw
- ¼ tsp minced garlic
- ¾ tbsp. apple cider vinegar
- ½ of a lime, juiced, zested

Seasoning:

- ¼ tsp paprika
- ¼ tsp salt
- 2 tbsp. avocado oil
- 1 tbsp. unsalted butter

Directions:

1. Prepare the marinade and for this, take a medium bowl, add vinegar, oil, garlic, paprika, salt, lime juice, and zest and stir until well mixed.

2. Cut chicken thighs into bite-size pieces, toss until well mixed, and marinate it in the refrigerator for 30 minutes.

3. Then take a skillet pan, place it over medium-high heat, add butter and marinated chicken pieces and cook for 8 minutes until golden brown and thoroughly cooked.

4. Serve chicken with coleslaw.

Nutrition:

- Net Carbohydrates: 1 g
- Protein: 9 g
- Fat: 12.8 g
- Calories: 157.3

Chicken Parmigiana

Preparation Time: 15 minutes

Cooking Time: 25 minutes

Servings: 2

Ingredients:

- 2 (6-oz.) grass-fed skinless, boneless chicken breasts
- 1 large organic egg, beaten
- 1/2 cup superfine blanched almond flour
- 1/4 cup Parmesan cheese, grated
- 1/2 tsp. dried parsley
- 1/2 tsp. paprika
- 1/2 tsp. garlic powder
- Salt and ground black pepper, as required
- 1/4 cup olive oil
- 1 cup sugar-free tomato sauce
- 5 oz. mozzarella cheese, thinly sliced
- 2 tbsp. fresh parsley, chopped

Directions:

1. Preheat your oven to 375°F.
2. Arrange one chicken breast between 2 pieces of parchment paper.
3. With a meat mallet, lb. chicken breast into a 1/2-inch thickness
4. Repeat with the remaining chicken breasts.
5. Add the beaten egg into a shallow dish.

6. Place the almond flour, Parmesan, parsley, spices, salt, and black pepper in another shallow dish, and mix well.

7. Dip chicken breasts into the whipped egg and then coat with the flour mixture.

8. Heat the oil in a deep wok over medium-high heat and fry the chicken breasts for about 3 minutes per side.

9. The chicken breasts must be transferred onto a paper towel-lined plate to drain.

10. At the bottom of a casserole, place about 1/2 cup of tomato sauce and spread evenly.

11. Arrange the chicken breasts over marinara sauce in a single layer.

12. Put sauce on top plus the mozzarella cheese slices.

13. Bake for about 20 minutes or until done completely.

14. Remove from the oven and serve hot with the garnishing of parsley.

Nutrition:

- Net Carbohydrates: 4.1g
- Protein: 15.1g
- Fat: 15.1g
- Calories: 398

Chicken Meatloaf Cups with Pancetta

Preparation Time: 15 minutes

Cooking Time: 30 minutes

Servings: 2

Ingredients:

- 2 tbsp. onion, chopped
- 1 tsp. garlic, minced
- 1-lb. ground chicken
- 2 oz. cooked pancetta, chopped
- 1 egg, beaten
- 1 tsp. mustard
- Salt and black pepper to taste
- 1/2 tsp. crushed red pepper flakes
- 1 tsp. dried basil
- 1/2 tsp. dried oregano
- 4 oz. cheddar cheese, cubed

Directions:

1. In a mixing bowl, mix mustard, onion, ground chicken, egg, bacon, and garlic. Season with oregano, red pepper, black pepper, basil, and salt.
2. Split the mixture into muffin cups—lower one cube of cheddar cheese into each meatloaf cup.
3. Close the top to cover the cheese.
4. Bake in the oven at 345°F for 20 minutes, or until the meatloaf cups become golden brown.

Nutrition:

- Net Carbohydrates: 3.9 g
- Protein: 11.4g
- Fat: 10.4g
- Calories: 231

Bell Pepper Eggs

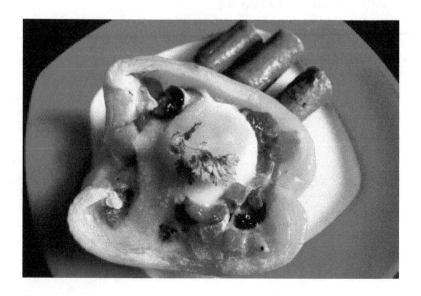

Preparation Time: 10 minutes

Cooking Time: 4 minutes

Servings: 2

Ingredients:

- 1 green bell pepper
- 2 eggs

Seasoning:

- 1 tsp coconut oil
- ¼ tsp salt
- ¼ tsp ground black pepper

Directions:

1. Prepare pepper rings, and for this, cut out two slices from the pepper, about ¼-inch, and reserve the remaining bell pepper for later use.

2. Take a skillet pan, place it over medium heat, grease it with oil, place pepper rings in it, and then crack an egg into each ring.

3. Season eggs with salt and black pepper, cook for 4 minutes, or until eggs have cooked to the desired level.

4. Transfer eggs to a plate and serve.

Nutrition:

- Net Carbohydrates: 1.7 g
- Protein: 7.2 g
- Fat: 8 g
- Calories: 110.5

Egg Butter

Preparation Time: 5 minutes

Cooking Time: 0 minutes

Servings: 2

Ingredients:

- 2 large eggs, hard-boiled
- 3-oz. unsalted butter
- ½ tsp dried oregano
- ½ tsp dried basil
- 2 leaves of iceberg lettuce

Seasoning:

- ½ tsp of sea salt
- ¼ tsp ground black pepper

Directions:

1. Peel the eggs, then chop them finely and place in a medium bowl.
2. Add remaining ingredients and stir well.
3. Serve egg butter wrapped in a lettuce leaf.

Nutrition:

- Net Carbohydrates: 0.2 g
- Protein: 3 g
- Fat: 16.5 g
- Calories: 159

VEGETABLES & SALADS

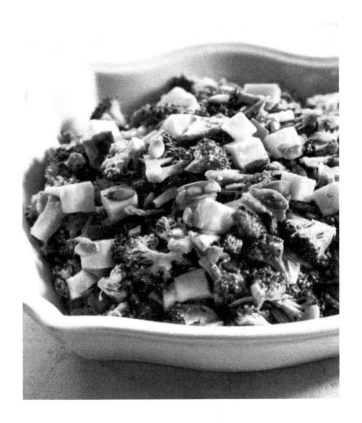

Blue Cheese and Bacon Kale Salad

Preparation Time: 10 minutes

Cooking Time: 10 minutes

Servings: 2

Ingredients:

- 4 bacon slices
- 2 cups stemmed and chopped fresh kale
- 1 tbsp. vinaigrette salad dressing (I use Primal Kitchen Greek Vinaigrette)
- Pinch pink Himalayan salt
- Pinch freshly ground black pepper
- ¼ cup pecans
- ¼ cup blue cheese crumbles

Directions:

1. In a medium skillet over medium-high heat, cook the bacon on both sides until crispy, about 8 minutes. Transfer the bacon to a paper towel-lined plate.

2. Meanwhile, in a large bowl, massage the kale with the vinaigrette for 2 minutes. Add the pink Himalayan salt and pepper. Let the kale sit while the bacon cooks, and it will get even softer.

3. Chop the bacon and pecans, and add them to the bowl. Sprinkle in the blue cheese.

4. Toss well to combine, portion onto two plates, and serve.

5. Chopped almonds can replace the chopped pecans.

Nutrition:

- Net Carbohydrates: 7g
- Protein: 16g
- Fat: 29g
- Calories: 353

Chopped Greek Salad

Preparation Time: 10 minutes

Cooking Time: 10 minutes

Servings: 2

Ingredients:

- 2 cups chopped romaine
- ½ cup halved grape tomatoes
- ¼ cup sliced black olives (like Kalamata)
- ¼ cup feta cheese crumbles
- 2 tbsp. vinaigrette salad dressing (I use Primal Kitchen Greek Vinaigrette)
- Pink Himalayan salt
- Freshly ground black pepper
- 1 tbsp. olive oil

Directions:

1. In a large bowl, combine the romaine, tomatoes, olives, feta cheese, and vinaigrette.
2. Season with pink Himalayan salt and pepper, drizzle with olive oil and toss to combine.
3. Divide the salad between two bowls and serve.
4. **Variations:**
5. With Greek salad, there are so many great flavors you can add:

6. Red onion or finely chopped cucumbers for additional crunch and freshness, and chopped pepperoncini for a zesty kick.

7. Finely chopped Genoa salami and pepperoni are good choices.

8. You could replace the feta cheese with goat cheese.

Nutrition:

- Net Carbohydrates: 3g
- Protein: 4g
- Fat: 19g
- Calories: 202

Mediterranean Cucumber Salad

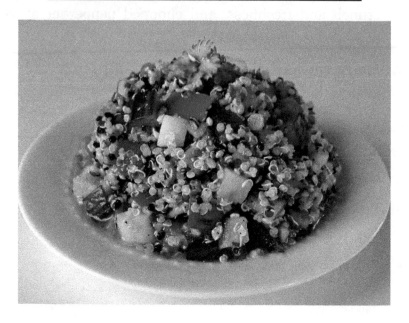

Preparation Time: 10 minutes

Cooking Time: 15 minutes

Servings: 2

Ingredients:

- 1 large cucumber, peeled and finely chopped
- ½ cup halved grape tomatoes
- ¼ cup halved black olives (I used Kalamata)
- ¼ cup crumbled feta cheese
- Pink Himalayan salt
- Freshly ground black pepper
- 2 tbsp. vinaigrette salad dressing (I use Primal Kitchen Greek Vinaigrette)

Directions:

1. In a large bowl, combine the cucumber, tomatoes, olives, and feta cheese—season with pink Himalayan salt and pepper. Add the dressing and toss to combine.

2. Divide the salad between two bowls and serve.

3. This salad can be eaten immediately, of course, but I think it is even better if you cover it with wrap and put it in the fridge to let the dressing marinate the salad ingredients for a few hours.

Nutrition:

- Net Carbohydrates: 4g
- Fat: 13g
- Protein: 4g
- Calories: 152

Avocado Egg Salad Lettuce Cups

Preparation Time: 15 minutes

Cooking Time: 15 minutes

Servings: 2

Ingredients:

- 4 large eggs
- 1 avocado halved
- Pink Himalayan salt
- Freshly ground black pepper
- ½ tsp. freshly squeezed lemon juice
- 4 butter lettuce cups washed and patted dry with paper towels or a clean dish towel
- 2 radishes, thinly sliced

Directions:

To make the hardboiled eggs:

1. In a medium saucepan, cover the eggs with water. Place over high heat and bring the water to a boil. Once it is boiling, turn off the heat, cover, and leave it on the burner for 10 to 12 minutes.
2. Remove the eggs with a slotted spoon and run them under cold water for 1 minute or submerge them in an ice bath.
3. Then gently tap the shells and peel. Run cold water over your hands as you remove the shells.

To make the egg salad:

1. In a medium bowl, chop the hardboiled eggs.

2. Add the avocado to the bowl and mash the flesh with a fork. Season with pink Himalayan salt and pepper, add the lemon juice and stir to combine.

3. Place the four lettuce cups on two plates. Top the lettuce cups with the egg salad and the slices of radish and serve.

Variations:

1. For this recipe, you can incorporate additional ingredients that you may have in your refrigerator or pantry:

2. Add a guacamole vibe to your egg salad with chopped jalapeño and red onion.

3. Chopped bacon adds appealing texture to your egg salad, or add slices of crisp bacon to your lettuce cups.

4. You could also use romaine hearts or baby cos lettuce.

Nutrition:

- Net Carbohydrates: 3g
- Protein: 15g
- Fat: 20g
- Calories: 258

VEGETARIAN

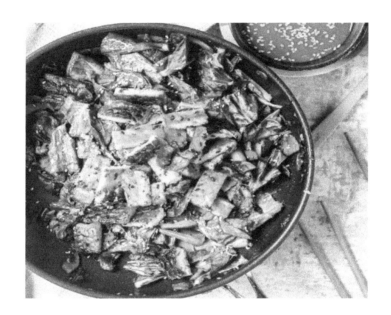

Baked Zucchini Gratin

Preparation Time: 25 minutes

Cooking Time: 30 minutes

Servings: 2

Ingredients:

- 1 large zucchini, cut into 1/4-inch-thick slices
- Pink Himalayan salt
- 1-oz. Brie cheese, rind trimmed off
- 1 tbsp. butter
- Freshly ground black pepper
- 1/3 cup shredded Gruyere cheese
- 1/4 cup crushed pork rinds

Directions:

1. Preheat the oven to 400°F.
2. When the zucchini has been "weeping" for about 30 minutes, in a small saucepan over medium-low heat, heat the Brie and butter, occasionally stirring, until the cheese melts.
3. The mixture is thoroughly combined for about 2 minutes.
4. Arrange the zucchini in an 8-inch baking dish, so the zucchini slices are overlapping a bit.
5. Season with pepper.
6. Pour the Brie mixture over the zucchini, and top with the shredded Gruyere cheese.
7. Sprinkle the crushed pork rinds over the top.

8. Bake for about 25 minutes, until the dish is boiling, and the top is nicely browned, and serve.

Nutrition:

- Net Carbohydrates: 2.2 g
- Protein: 5.1g
- Fat: 11.5g
- Calories: 324

Veggie Greek Moussaka

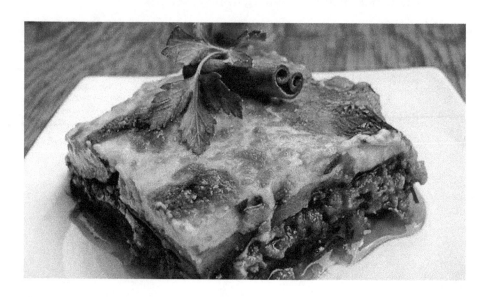

Preparation Time: 20 minutes

Cooking Time: 30 minutes

Servings: 2

Ingredients:

- 2 large eggplants, cut into strips
- 1 cup diced celery
- 1 cup diced carrots
- 1 small white onion, chopped
- 2 eggs
- 1 tsp. olive oil
- 3 cups grated Parmesan
- 1 cup ricotta cheese

- 3 cloves garlic, minced
- 2 tsp. Italian seasoning blend
- Salt to taste

Sauce:

- 1 1/2 cups heavy cream
- 1/4 cup butter, melted
- 1 cup grated mozzarella cheese
- 2 tsp. Italian seasoning
- 3/4 cup almond flour

Directions:

1. Preheat the oven to 350°F.
2. Lay the eggplant strips, sprinkle with salt, and let sit there to exude liquid. Heat olive oil heat and sauté the onion, celery, garlic, and carrots for 5 minutes.
3. Mix the eggs, 1 cup of Parmesan cheese, ricotta cheese, and salt in a bowl; set aside.
4. Pour the heavy cream into a pot and bring to heat over a medium fire while continually stirring.
5. Stir in the remaining Parmesan cheese and one tsp. of Italian seasoning. Turn the heat off and set it aside.
6. To lay the moussaka, spread a small amount of the sauce at the bottom of the baking dish.
7. Pat dry the eggplant strips and make a single layer on the sauce.

8. A layer of ricotta cheese must be spread on the eggplants, sprinkle some veggies on it, and repeat everything

9. In a small bowl, evenly mix the melted butter, almond flour, and one tsp. of Italian seasoning.

10. Spread the top of the moussaka layers with it, and sprinkle the top with mozzarella cheese.

11. Bake for 25 minutes until the cheese is slightly burned. Slice the moussaka and serve warm.

Nutrition:

- Net Carbohydrates: 3.1 g
- Protein: 5.9g
- Fat: 15.1g
- Calories: 398

Gouda Cauliflower Casserole

Preparation Time: 15 minutes

Cooking Time: 15 minutes

Servings: 2

Ingredients:

- 2 heads cauliflower, cut into florets
- 1/3 cup butter, cubed
- 2 tbsp. melted butter
- 1 white onion, chopped
- Salt and black pepper to taste
- 1/4 almond milk
- 1/2 cup almond flour
- 1 1/2 cups grated gouda cheese

Directions:

1. Preheat the oven to 350°F and put the cauliflower florets in a large microwave-safe bowl.
2. Sprinkle with a bit of water and steam in the microwave for 4 to 5 minutes.
3. Melt the 1/3 cup of butter in a saucepan over medium heat and sauté the onion for 3 minutes.
4. Add the cauliflower, season with salt and black pepper, and mix in almond milk. Simmer for 3 minutes.
5. Mix the remaining melted butter with almond flour.

6. Stir into the cauliflower as well as half of the cheese. Sprinkle the top with the remaining cheese and bake for 10 minutes until the cheese has melted and golden brown.

7. Plate the bake and serve with salad.

Nutrition:

- Net Carbohydrates: 4.1 g
- Protein: 10g
- Fat: 9.4g
- Calories: 349

SNACKS, SIDES & SAUCES

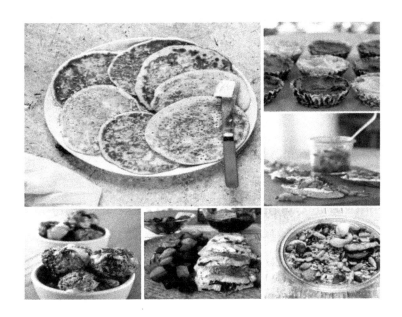

Cheesy Mushroom Slices

Preparation Time: 8-10 minutes

Cooking Time: 15 minutes

Servings: 2

Ingredients:

- 2 cup mushrooms
- 2 eggs
- ¾ cup almond flour
- ½ cup cheddar cheese
- 2 tbsps. Butter
- ½ tsp. Pepper
- ¼ tsp. salt

Directions:

1. Process chopped mushrooms in a food processor, then add eggs, almond flour, and cheddar cheese.
2. Put salt and pepper, then pour melted butter into the food processor. Transfer.
3. Warm-up an Air Fryer to 375°F (191°C).
4. Put the loaf pan on the Air Fryer's rack, then cook for 15 minutes. Slice and serve.

Nutrition:

- Net Carbohydrates: 4.4g
- Protein: 10.4g
- Fat: 34.6g
- Calories: 365

Asparagus Fries

Preparation Time: 10 minutes

Cooking Time: 10 minutes

Servings: 2

Ingredients:

- 10 organic asparagus spears
- 1 tbsp. organic roasted red pepper
- ¼ cup almond flour
- ½ tsp. garlic powder
- ½ tsp. smoked paprika
- 2 tbsp. parsley
- ½ cup parmesan cheese, and full-fat
- 2 organic eggs
- 3 tbsp. mayonnaise, full-fat

Directions:

1. Warm-up oven to 425 degrees F.
2. Process cheese in a food processor, add garlic and parsley and pulse for 1 minute.
3. Add almond flour, pulse for 30 seconds, transfer, and put paprika.
4. Whisk eggs into a shallow dish.
5. Dip asparagus spears into the egg batter, then coat with parmesan mixture and place it on a baking sheet. Bake in the oven for 10 minutes.

6. Put the mayonnaise in a bowl, add red pepper and whisk, then chill. Serve with prepared dip.

Nutrition:

- Net Carbohydrates: 5.5 g
- Protein: 19.1 g
- Fat: 33.4 g
- Calories: 453

Guacamole

Preparation Time: 10 minutes

Cooking Time: 0 minutes

Servings: 2

Ingredients:

- 2 organic avocados pitted
- 1/3 organic red onion
- 1 organic jalapeño
- 1/2 tsp. salt
- 1/2 tsp. ground pepper
- 2 tbsp. tomato salsa
- 1 tbsp. lime juice
- 1/2 organic cilantro

Directions:

1. Slice the avocado flesh horizontally and vertically.
2. Mix in onion, jalapeno, and lime juice in a bowl.
3. Put salt and black pepper, add salsa and mix. Fold in cilantro and serve.

Nutrition:

- Net Carbohydrates: 0.5 g
- Protein: 0.23 g
- Fat: 1.4 g
- Calories: 16.5

Zucchini Noodles

Preparation Time: 5 minutes

Cooking Time: 6 minutes

Servings: 2

Ingredients:

- 2 zucchinis, spiralized into noodles
- 2 tbsp. butter, unsalted
- 1 ½ tbsp. garlic
- 3/4 cup parmesan cheese
- ½ tsp. sea salt
- 1/4 tsp. ground black pepper
- 1/4 tsp. red chili flakes

Directions:

1. Sauté butter and garlic for 1 minute.
2. Put zucchini noodles, cook for 5 minutes, then put salt and black pepper.
3. Transfer then top with cheese and sprinkle with red chili flakes. Serve.

Nutrition:

- Net Carbohydrates: 2.3 g
- Protein: 5 g
- Fat: 26.1 g
- Calories: 298

DESSERTS

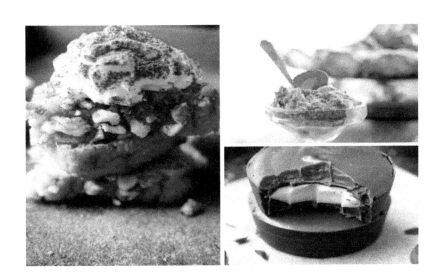

Chocolate Mousse

Preparation Time: 15 minutes

Cooking Time: 0 minutes

Servings: 2

Ingredients:

- 8.5 oz. mascarpone cheese
- 2 tbsp. cocoa powder, unsweetened
- 1 tbsp. of a sweetener
- 1 tsp. vanilla extract

Directions:

1. Place mousse in serving cups, serve and enjoy.

Nutrition:

- Net Carbohydrates: 2 g
- Protein: 4 g
- Fat: 27 g
- Calories: 286

Pomegranate Pudding

Preparation Time: 15 minutes

Cooking Time: 10 minutes

Servings: 2

Ingredients:

- 14.5 oz. coconut milk
- ½ cup pomegranate seeds
- 3 tbsp. raw honey
- 2 tbsp. coconut oil
- 1 tbsp. vanilla extract
- 1 packet gelatin, unflavored

Directions:

1. Stir in the honey with coconut milk and vanilla extract.
2. Cook coconut mixture until it starts to boil, then gently add gelatin until completely melted.
3. Stir in the pomegranate seeds and pour the mixture into serving cups, then refrigerate for 4 hours.
4. Serve the coconut pudding and enjoy.

Nutrition:

- Net Carbohydrates: 16.5 g
- Protein: 8.6 g
- Fat: 31.3 g
- Calories: 386

Berry Lemon Cake

Preparation Time: 15 minutes

Cooking Time: 30 minutes

Servings: 2

Ingredients:

- 1/2 cup fresh blueberries
- 1/2 cup coconut flour
- 1/3 cup coconut milk
- 1/3 cup raw honey
- 3 eggs, beaten
- 2 ½ tbsp. coconut oil, melted
- 2 tbsp. fresh lemon juice
- 1 tbsp. lemon zest, grated
- 1 tsp. lemon extract
- 1 tsp. apple cider vinegar
- 1/2 tsp. baking soda
- Salt

Directions:

1. Preheat the oven to 350 F.
2. Mix the apple cider with baking soda in a small bowl.
3. Mix the baking soda mix with coconut oil, lemon juice, and zest, lemon extract, coconut flour and honey, coconut milk, eggs, and a pinch of salt until no lumps are found, then fold in the berries.

4. Pour the batter into a greased baking dish, then bake it for 30 mins.

Nutrition:

- Net Carbohydrates: 12.6 g
- Fat: 13.4 g
- Protein: 3.5 g
- Calories: 203

Keto Frosty

Preparation Time: 45 minutes

Cooking Time: 0 minutes

Servings: 2

Ingredients:

- 1 ½ cups heavy whipping cream
- 2 tbsp. cocoa powder (unsweetened)
- 3 tbsp. Swerve
- 1 tsp. pure vanilla extract
- Salt to taste

Directions:

1. In a bowl, combine all the ingredients.
2. Use a hand mixer and beat until you see stiff peaks forming.
3. Place the mixture in a Ziploc bag.
4. Freeze for 35 minutes.
5. Serve in bowls or dishes.

Nutrition:

- Total Carbohydrate 2.9g
- Protein 1.4g
- Fat 17g
- Calories 164

Keto Shake

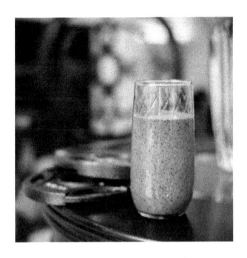

Preparation Time: 15 minutes

Cooking Time: 0 minutes

Servings: 2

Ingredients:

- ¾ cup almond milk
- ½ cup ice
- 2 tbsp. almond butter
- 2 tbsp. cocoa powder (unsweetened)
- 2 tbsp. Swerve
- 1 tbsp. chia seeds
- 2 tbsp. hemp seeds
- ½ tbsp. vanilla extract
- Salt to taste

Directions:

1. Blend all the ingredients in a food processor.
2. Chill in the refrigerator before serving.

Nutrition:

- Total Carbohydrate 3.6g
- Protein 1.6g
- Fat 9.5g
- Calories 104

DRINKS

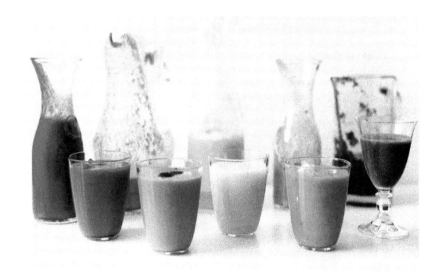

Kiwi Coconut Smoothie

Preparation Time: 5 minutes

Cooking Time: 0 minutes

Servings: 2

Ingredients:

- 2 kiwis, pulp scooped
- 1 tbsp. xylitol
- 4 ice cubes
- 2 cups unsweetened coconut milk
- 1 cup of coconut yogurt
- Mint leaves to garnish

Directions:

1. Process the kiwis, xylitol, coconut milk, yogurt, and ice cubes in a blender until smooth, for about 3 minutes.
2. Transfer to serving glasses, garnish with mint leaves, and serve.

Nutrition:

- Net Carbohydrates: 1.2 g
- Protein: 3.2g
- Fat: 1.2g
- Calories: 298

Avocado-Coconut Shake

Preparation Time: 5 minutes

Cooking Time: 0 minutes

Servings: 2

Ingredients:

- 3 cups coconut milk, chilled
- 1 avocado, pitted, peeled, sliced
- 2 tbsp. erythritol
- Coconut cream for topping

Directions:

1. Combine coconut milk, avocado, and erythritol, into the smoothie maker, and blend for 1 minute to smooth. Pour the drink into serving glasses, add some coconut cream on top of them, and garnish with mint leaves. Serve immediately.

Nutrition:

- Net Carbohydrates: 0.4 g
- Protein: 3.1g
- Fat: 6.4g
- Calories: 301

Blueberry Tofu Smoothie

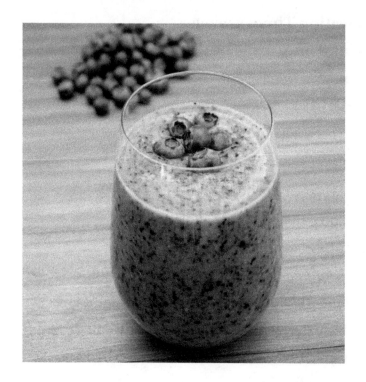

Preparation Time: 15 minutes

Cooking Time: 0 minutes

Servings: 2

Ingredients:

- 6 oz. of silken tofu
- 1 medium banana
- 2/3 cups of soy milk
- 1 cup of frozen or fresh blueberries (divided)
- 1 tbsp. of honey
- 2-3 ice cubes (optional)

Directions:

1. Drain the silken tofu to remove the excess water (silken tofu as a high-water content)

2. Peele and slice the banana. Place the sliced banana on a baking sheet and freeze them. This process usually takes up to 15 minutes. This helps to make the smoothie thicker.

3. Get a blender. Blend the banana, tofu, and soy milk. This usually takes up to 30 seconds.

4. Add 1/2 cup of the blueberries to the banana, tofu, and soymilk. Then blend it until it is very smooth.

5. Put the remaining blueberries. Add honey and ice cubes. Blend it until it is well combined.

6. Serve and enjoy.

Nutrition:

- Net Carbohydrates: 2.7 g
- Protein: 12.1g
- Fat: 9.5g
- Calories: 312

Bulletproof Coffee

Preparation Time: 5 minutes

Cooking Time: 0 minutes

Servings: 2

Ingredients:

- 1 1/2 cups hot coffee
- 2 tbsp. MCT oil powder or Bulletproof Brain Octane Oil
- 2 tbsp. butter or ghee

Directions:

1. Pour the hot coffee into the blender.
2. Add the oil powder and butter, and blend until thoroughly mixed and frothy.
3. Pour into a large mug and enjoy.

Nutrition:

- Net Carbohydrates: 1.2 g
- Protein: 2.3g
- Fat: 9.4g
- Calories: 245

Morning Berry-Green Smoothie

Preparation Time: 15 minutes

Cooking Time: 0 minutes

Servings: 2

Ingredients:

- 1 avocado, pitted and sliced
- 3 cups mixed blueberries and strawberries
- 2 cups unsweetened almond milk
- 6 tbsp. heavy cream
- 2 tsp. erythritol
- 1 cup of ice cubes
- 1/3 cup nuts and seeds mix

Directions:

1. Combine the avocado slices, blueberries, strawberries, almond milk, heavy cream, erythritol, ice cubes, nuts, and seeds in a smoothie maker; blend in high-speed until smooth and uniform.
2. Pour the smoothie into drinking glasses and serve immediately.

Nutrition:

- Net Carbohydrates: 1.4 g
- Protein: 2g
- Fat: 5.1g
- Calories: 290

CONCLUSION

Thank you for reading all this book!

The ketogenic diet is not just a diet –it is a healthy, weight-reducing way of life. This diet can help you to not only lose weight but control blood pressure, increase mental focus, boost energy, and improve overall health. Keto success is achieved by following low-carbohydrate principles.

Developing and implementing a Keto-friendly diet plan will help to ensure that you are eating nutrient-rich foods while eliminating calorie-dense foods that hold no nutritional value.

You have already taken a step towards your improvement.

Best wishes!

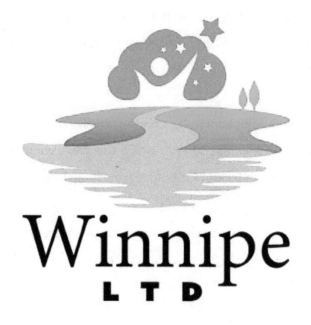

Winnipe
L T D